Using Mindfulness and Positive Focus to Ease Depression, Anxiety and Pain

A 30-Day Journal with Exercises to Power Your Journey To Inner Peace

Marcia A. Hillary, PhD

DISCLAIMER

The exercises and suggestions presented in this book are generic. They are not therapy, and they are not intended to serve as a replacement for appropriate medical or behavioral health treatment. Anyone with a medical or behavioral health problem is encouraged to consult their treating health care provider(s) and discuss the suitability of these exercises, as well as any modifications that may be necessary for their specific needs and circumstances.

First published by Dog Ear Publishing
4010 W. 86th Street, Ste H
Indianapolis, IN 46268
www.dogearpublishing.net

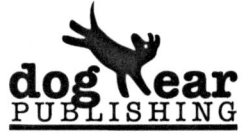

ISBN: 978-1-4575-1409-8

This book is printed on acid-free paper.

Printed in the United States of America

*This book is dedicated to Nicky, who radiates love and demonstrates
the ability to live fully in each moment*

and to you, wherever you are at this moment on your journey to inner peace.

CONTENTS

ABOUT THIS JOURNAL

This 30-day journal focuses on mindfulness and a positive attitude. Negativity is all around us, and it can be easy for all of us to fall prey to it. If you currently are feeling depressed or anxious, or if you experience physical pain, you probably are an expert about focusing on negative thoughts, feelings, and experiences. I hope you learn a different approach to life from this journal. I am part of the "movement" that focuses on the positive, which helps the positive become more of our way of life. This journal can accompany your work with me or with another therapist, or you can use this journal on your own as you approach your life in a mindful manner. Please be mindful of the disclosure earlier in this journal. This journal isn't therapy and isn't intended to be a substitute for appropriate behavioral health or physical health intervention.

An article in the <u>American Psychologist</u> (Munoz, Beardslee, & Leykin, 2012) titled "Major Depression Can Be Prevented" grabbed my attention. The article discussed the 2009 Institute of Medicine report (National Research Council & Institute of Medicine, 2009) on the prevention of mental, emotional and behavioral disorders which provided evidence that major depression can be prevented. How's that for raising eyebrows! How's that for thinking positively!

You'll notice that I'm interested only in your positive thoughts and feelings, and your feelings and thoughts of gratitude. Your positive thoughts are worthy of your focus and attention. Your negative thoughts are the weeds in the beautiful garden of your life. The negative thoughts (weeds) are there, but they aren't the main crop. I invite you to spend most of your time and energy focusing on what you want to cultivate in the garden of your life: positive thoughts, positive feelings, pleasant sensations. Weeds may keep popping up, but with your proper attention, some weeding and some healthy nutrients (the equivalent of sun, water, and organic fertilizer), I hope your garden and your life will be filled with beauty and inner peace!

This is a journal for you to use on the next month of your life's journey. I encourage you to participate for the full 30 days, and then you may decide to continue on your charted course, or to modify the journal to fit your specific needs. This journal is meant as a guide to accompany your self awareness process, which you might also call your journey to inner peace. I'm on that journey, too. My hope is that in this next month you begin to pay attention to your body in a new, positive way; that you begin to experience mindfulness more often; that you demonstrate a more positive outlook about yourself and your life . . . There are unlimited positive possibilities for this next month of your life!

To participate fully in all the exercises in this journal you could easily spend two or three hours daily. Some of you have that amount of time readily available, while many won't. I encourage you to spend at least 45 minutes daily with the exercises in this journal. That's about the length of a typical session of psychotherapy, and much longer than you'd typically spend talking with your physician. Over the course of the next 30 days, I encourage you to do all the exercises at least a few times, and you'll probably select several that are most meaningful for you. I hope you'll continue with those exercises indefinitely.

There are many books on mindfulness and on breathing. Some of my favorites are *Full Catastrophe Living* (1990) and *Wherever You Go There You Are* (1994) by Jon Kabat-Zinn, PhD and *Conscious Breathing* (1995) by Gay Hendricks, PhD.

Mindfulness refers to paying attention to the present moment, without judging that moment as good or bad, painful or pain free, positive or negative. How often are we lost in our thoughts or multi-tasking while we drive our vehicle, take a walk, eat, respond to email, etc. Paying attention to the present moment allows us to fully live in the present moment. The present moment is the only moment we have right now — we don't know how many future moments we'll have, and if we're busy anticipating the future (by worrying or by eagerly looking forward to something) we miss the gift of our present moment. Yes, we can choose to furnish the present moment with worry, or with angry thoughts, or with plans to "get even" with someone; my hope is that we'll choose a more positive way to embrace the gift of that moment.

For those of us who refer to our thoughts as emanating from our "mind," we can realize that thoughts produced "mindlessly" often prompt over-eating, anger, jealousy, sadness, depression or anxiety. Thoughts produced "mindlessly" could also produce continual happiness or joy, but in our society few of us think "happy thoughts" continually without conscious attention. We tend to dwell on what produces pain, fear, anger, jealousy, and other negative feelings.

Although you may begin this journal with an experience of physical and/or emotional pain, you'll notice that the positive aspects of your life are emphasized. Whatever we think about, whatever we dwell on, whatever we ruminate about — that is what usually happens, or continues to happen. When all we think about is negative, we usually get a result of more negative. You've probably been thinking about your personal experience of discontent before buying this journal, so you're already an expert on the negative. You don't need me to teach you about that!

If you're ready to get off the "pain train" (depression, anxiety, chronic pain, etc.) and you're ready to learn some different techniques, and you're willing to *practice* those techniques for at least 30 days (that's just one month of your life!) you may find yourself humming a different tune in 30 days. I encourage you to adopt an open mind, and an open heart.

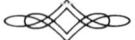

HOW TO GET THE MOST BENEFIT FROM THIS JOURNAL

It's my privilege to help you get started on this 30-day journey. I'll start with some "how to" information. By putting this information in its own section at the beginning, you'll know where to look for it and it won't bog you down each day. Be sure you read this section thoroughly, and do review it from time to time.

Each day I encourage you to participate in several exercises. Even if you don't like an exercise initially, I encourage you to continue with it for several days and find out if you have the same opinion later. Sometimes we grow to appreciate tasks we didn't like initially. At the end of the 30 days, you can choose to continue any or all of the exercises in this journal and begin to make them part of your daily lifestyle. You can continue doing some or all of the exercises without charting daily, but journaling your experience may help you to be mindful of that experience.

One of the basic premises of workbooks and programs on stress management, meditation, relaxation techniques, or any other personal growth tools is that we can only realize the benefits of the program after we've practiced those techniques regularly over a period of time. Reading about techniques just isn't enough. Personal experience is crucial. Here in this journal you'll be able to record your experiences daily. This helps you prove to yourself that you did the exercises, and provides a day-by-day record of your journey. I encourage you to limit any reviewing of your journey initially. Stay in the moment. Let at least two weeks go by before you review what you wrote on the first days of your journey.

Regular, persistent practice is important. When you practice regularly, you really learn how to perform each exercise so that you can do it without referring back to instructions. Regular practice is also necessary in order to form a habit. No one can make these exercises part of their daily life style without engaging in them regularly; daily would be ideal, of course, and that's the intention of this journal. Persistent practice over time can make a huge difference in your life.

Is there a "best" time to do these journal exercises? Any time during the day or evening is better than not doing the exercises at all! A benefit of journaling in the morning is that it helps jump-start your day in a positive way. A benefit of journaling in the evening is that you may set the stage for peaceful, restful sleep. Either, or both, can be valuable, as well as any time in between morning and evening.

You may be thinking that you don't have enough time to do these exercises daily. The exercises do take some time. They usually take longer when you're just learning them, and in a different way, they can take more time when you're engaging in them whole-heartedly. That usually means you're benefiting from that exercise! Can you spare 45 - 60 minutes daily to feel better about yourself and your life? Right now, this might seem like a huge effort; I hope you come to regard these exercises as a precious gift to yourself.

You are cordially invited to embark on a 30-day journey during which You may learn:

to become more aware of more parts of your physical body

to differentiate your inner world from your external world

to focus on positive elements of your life

TO INCLUDE GRATITUDE IN YOUR DAILY THOUGHTS

to become mindful of your breathing (and maybe other things too)

to experience moments of inner peace (remember that life is a series of moments)

This journey begins at

_____
your address

at _____
time you choose

EXERCISES AND MEDITATIONS

So, you've accepted the invitation and you're ready to start. The instructions to all the exercises and meditations in this journal are in this section. Refer to these instructions occasionally to be sure you are staying on course. There's plenty of space for you to write in this journal each day.

SELF RATING I

To start each day's journal exercises, take a moment to rate your current position on four components of yourself. Rate quickly without thinking too much. Rate your immediate impression or awareness.

> *physiological:* your current level of physical comfort or relaxation
> *mental:* the quality of your current thoughts and mental preoccupation
> *emotional:* your feelings about your physical body, your thoughts, your life
> *spiritual:* your experience of connection with God/Goddess/Higher Self

The rating scale ranges from 1 to 7. Rate yourself on each of the four components.

1: totally uncomfortable; I experience no comfort or inner peace
2: a tiny amount of comfort or inner peace; I'm mostly aware of discomfort or disconnectedness
3: comfort or inner peace is somewhat overshadowed by discomfort or disconnectedness
4: my comfort or inner peace is balanced evenly with tension or disconnectedness
5: comfort or inner peace is slightly more noticeable than tension or disconnectedness
6: comfort or inner peace is predominant; I feel quite relaxed and peaceful
7: I'm totally relaxed and peaceful

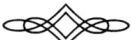

BODY SCAN

Our society is pre-occupied with bodies — our body shape and size, the ideal bodies portrayed in many ads, the body we used to have before pain or extra weight moved in. Some people don't accept their body, or don't feel comfortable in their body. Some people experience physical pain, and others experience emotional pain that sometimes includes physical discomfort. Some people dislike being touched because they don't want to feel their body. Thinking about our physical body often leads to judging it, usually in a negative way. Regardless of how our body feels, and without judging it as *too XYZ* or *not enough ABC*, it is important to actually become mindful of our body whatever it looks or feels like, without judging it.

This body scan exercise or meditation may help you develop mindful concentration while you focus your attention on your physical body, part by part. You can accomplish this body scan in five minutes, but I encourage you to spend 30 - 45 minutes each day (twice daily if you choose).

I invite you to have a sense of curiosity each time you practice this exercise. Over time, you may realize that your body is different each time you do this exercise, even when you practice twice in the same day.

Forget about using this exercise to change something, or to get someplace else. That's usually called "striving." It's common, even human, to want to change from feeling depressed or anxious or painful to feeling peaceful, but that focus on wanting to change probably won't help you change. It's more likely to keep you focused on whatever pain you are in. So, I encourage you to be where you are now, practice without any goal of getting somewhere else, and suspend judging yourself. During this exercise, be who you are.

If you experience difficulty feeling part of your body, or if you are so overwhelmed by physical pain in some part of your body that you can't concentrate on any other part of your body, then that is your awareness at that moment. "I don't feel anything" can be your experience of your toes. If intense neck pain interferes with your ability to pay attention to your toes or fingers, shift to a different position first to see if that helps. If pain continually calls your attention to your neck (or anywhere else), be aware of that discomfort and keep returning your attention to the exercise. Be as open and receptive as possible as you move your attention through this exercise. Perhaps you will learn to move through the most intense discomfort, to be open to all the sensations you experience at whatever level of intensity, to watch the sensations, breathe through the sensations, and let them go as you move on with the exercise.

On rare occasions, people experience flashbacks of prior physically or emotionally painful experiences which they had forgotten or repressed. If this happens to you, first, keep breathing. That event(s) that you suddenly remember is (are) over. You survived. You can discuss this memory with your therapist. Keep breathing. While focusing on this painful event can make it difficult to focus mindfully on the present moment, it's also very important to process this memory in therapy. If you aren't already working with a therapist, I encourage you to start working with a therapist. Keep breathing. If you experience any thought of self harm or suicide as you recall the painful event, take immediate emergency steps to protect yourself. If you are physically alone, find someone to stay with you or someone you can stay with. See your therapist on an emergency basis, call the nearest psychiatric hospital (they are open 24/7), call a suicide prevention hot line, call 911, etc. As terrifying or overwhelming as your memory may be, remember that it's a memory of something you have already gotten through. You can get help in processing the memory. Keep breathing. Focus on your breathing even as you take the steps to get to a place of safety. You are important. Your life has meaning.

When doing the body scan, a key point is to maintain your awareness throughout the exercise from a place of detachment. Witness your breath, witness each body part as you scan from your toes to your head. Being fully present in each moment and with each breath is important. Being present in each moment, in each breath, is being mindful. This mindfulness can help you heal whatever needs healing.

If you are missing a body part due to surgery or otherwise, you can still participate in this exercise. When you reach the part of your body that is no longer physically present, breathe into the space where that part was. From the perspective of energy, that part is still present, although not physically. Then move on to the next area of your body.

To begin the body scan, lie down comfortably, or at least as comfortably as possible, on your back. Use a foam pad or a sleeping bag, if you desire. You can lie on your bed as long as you don't fall asleep; your intention is to remain awake and present with each breath. Cover yourself with a blanket if necessary.

Allow your eyes to close gently. Notice your abdomen rise and fall with each breath. For a few breaths, notice what it's like to feel your whole body.

Now you'll start with the full body scan. Attend to the toes of your left foot. Feel those toes. Imagine feeling your toes. Imagine breathing right into your toes, and imagine breathing out from these toes. This can take awhile; many of us forget to use our imagination for positive thinking and use it only for worrying. It's OK to to use your imagination for positive purposes. Breathe. In and out. Breathe into the toes of your left foot. Breathe out from the toes of your left foot. You are likely to get better at this with practice, just as you improved your ability to ride a bike with practice.

Feel any sensations in your toes, and if you don't feel anything, that's OK. In that case, what you're feeling right now is "not feeling anything here now."

When you are ready to leave the toes, take a slightly deeper breath and imagine your toes dissolving as you exhale. Keep breathing in and out, and move your attention to the sole of your left foot, the heel of your left foot, the top of your left foot, your left ankle —- breathing into that body part and breathing out from that body part. Notice any sensations you experience. Notice any thoughts or feelings you experience. Keep returning your focus to your breath. Focus on each body part and move on to another body part.

After your left foot, focus your attention on the toes of your right foot, then the sole, heel, top of your right foot, right ankle. As your attention wanders, bring it back to your breath and whatever body part you're on.

After your feet, you can focus on the parts of both legs simultaneously or you can focus on each part of your left leg and then focus on the parts of your right leg. Whichever you choose, keep moving up your body, focusing your attention on your breath moving into and out of each body part —- your pelvic girdle, your abdomen, your heart, your lungs, your spine, all the way to your head. You can imagine the parts of each arm separately, or the parts of both arms simultaneously. If you think a lot, be sure to pay attention to your breath going into your head and out from your head.

If you experience pain or discomfort, you might imagine breathing in and out of that body part through the pain or discomfort, just like breathing on a foggy day when you can't see clearly. Or, you can breathe right into the pain/discomfort itself. As weird or difficult as it may sound, you can breathe or imagine breathing right into the pain/discomfort itself. I discourage ignoring pain altogether, and I really discourage gritting your teeth to endure pain. There have been experiments showing that actually tuning into the sensations of pain is more effective at reducing pain than distracting yourself from the pain. These are my suggestions. They have been used successfully by others. They may work for you, too. But remember that you are the expert on the particular pain you experience, and new research on pain is published almost daily.

If you fall asleep each time you do the body scan exercise, you may be sleep deprived, and your body may be catching up on the sleep it needs. Can you make adequate sleep time a priority? Falling asleep each time you do this exercise may also indicate that you feel safe and secure enough during the exercise to sleep. You may also do this exercise with your eyes open, paying attention to your breath.

This body scan exercise or meditation can take up to 45 minutes. I encourage taking that full amount of time, if possible. However, take at least 20 minutes for this exercise, and be sure you are focusing on your breath. Even if you spend only 20 minutes on this exercise, a little time is usually an improvement over no time! It may take longer for you to notice benefits if you have just five or ten minutes to practice. Just stay with it.

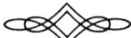

AWARENESS (INTERNAL/EXTERNAL)
This exercise may help you become aware of different parts of your body, and this exercise can help you learn to differentiate what's going on inside your body from what is going on outside your body.

Your breath is important. You might remind yourself "be mindful of my breath" as you engage in this exercise. If you experience an unpleasant sensation, thought or feeling, you can notice it and keep focusing on the exercise. If the sensation/thought/feeling is very uncomfortable, you can use your breath to enter it (just as was discussed during the body scan exercise). If the sensation/thought/feeling is severely disturbing and especially if you experience thoughts of self harm or suicide, stop the exercise immediately. Breathe. You have several options, as you did during the body scan exercise. You can discuss the sensation/thought/feeling with your therapist. While focusing on this sensation/thought/feeling can make it difficult to focus mindfully on the present moment, it's also very important to process this in therapy. If you aren't already working with a therapist, I encourage you to start working with one. Keep breathing. If you experience any thought of self harm or suicide, take immediate emergency steps to protect yourself. If you are physically alone, find someone to stay with you or someone you can stay with. See your therapist on an emergency basis, call the nearest psychiatric hospital (they are open 24/7), call a suicide prevention hot line, call 911, etc. As terrifying or overwhelming as the sensation/thought/ feeling may be, you can get through this. You can get help. Keep breathing. Focus on your breathing even as you take the steps to get to a place of safety. Remember, you are important. Your life has meaning.

To perform the awareness exercise, sit comfortably. Loosen any tight clothing if necessary. Eyes can be open or closed. If you leave your eyes open, gaze at one place and allow your eyes to be "soft" and unfocused, as often occurs during daydreaming when your eyes are open but your attention is focused elsewhere from whatever your eyes are looking at.

Focus your attention first on the world outside of you, your external world. Say aloud or silently five things you are currently aware of, beginning each sentence with "I am aware of." For example, "I am aware of a dog barking. I am aware of the car that just drove past my house. I am aware of the vase of flowers on the table. I am aware of the dirty spot on the carpet. I am aware of the rain on the windows." Notice that there is no judgment here; we're focused on awareness.

Next, focus your attention on your inner world, the sensations in your body. Say aloud or silently five things you are aware of regarding your current inner world. Start each sentence with "I am aware of." For example, "I am aware of my stuffy nose. I am aware of my right ankle itching. I am aware of discomfort in my lower back. I am aware of feeling tired. I am aware of feeling nervous about my appointment with my doctor this afternoon."

For a few minutes, shuttle back and forth between your awareness of your external world and your awareness of your internal world. Notice whatever you notice. Focus on your external world, and then notice your awareness of your internal world.

This exercise can help you distinguish what's you from what is not you. In other words, you can learn to distinguish between your outer world and your inner world. If you take in so much of your outer world that you notice it causes tension in your inner world or even that it seems like the outer world is your inner world, you can then decide what to do about that. You can't change anything unless you first become aware of it.

You can practice this exercise for a few minutes throughout each day. For example, you can do this exercise while you're in line at the grocery store, or while you're waiting for an appointment.

Remember to breathe. Note any recurring themes, or anything else that you notice from this exercise. You can jot that in your journal.

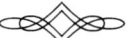

EATING A RAISIN (substitute a strawberry or shelled walnut if you prefer)
Once you have a raisin, strawberry or shelled walnut on a table in front of you, allow at least five minutes for this exercise. Observe your chosen object. See it, touch it, smell it. Is there a sound when you touch it? Observe it thoroughly. Focus on your object, not the clock. Keep observing. Keep studying your object. Only when it seems that you have learned all that you could possibly learn from your observation, consider placing the raisin (strawberry, walnut) in your mouth. Study your thought about putting the object in your mouth. Did you begin salivating when you started to think about placing the object in your mouth? Then go ahead and place the object in your mouth. Keep noticing: texture, taste, salivation. Are you comparing this raisin (strawberry, walnut) to other raisins (strawberries, walnuts) you've encountered previously? Chew, taste, notice, swallow, notice. When you feel complete with this exercise, notice the time. How long did you devote to this exercise? Were there extraneous thoughts? Feelings? Memories? Jot some notes of your experience in your journal. If your attention was totally focused on your chosen object and your experience with that object, you were practicing mindfulness. You were purposefully paying attention to the present moment.

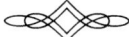

MINDFULNESS MEDITATION
Find someplace comfortable (but not so comfortable that you'll fall asleep) where you can sit with your back reasonably straight. Close your eyes if you want to reduce visual distractions, or leave them open. Breathe. In and out, through your nose. Pay attention to your breathing. In and out. Feel the air as you inhale, feel the air going into your nose, notice how far into your lungs the air goes, notice the air moving out of your body. Is there a different quality to your inhales than your exhales? Is one easier than the other? Is one freer than the other? *Just notice.* Keep breathing. Thoughts will show up, but gently focus on your breathing. Thoughts will keep showing up. Keep returning your attention gently to your breath. You may suddenly find yourself thinking about something you never would have paid attention to, except that now you're quiet, so suddenly you're having that thought. Just notice it, and return your attention gently to your breath. Notice your breath. In and out. That's it. Do this for as long as you like. This is mindfulness meditation. Although 45 minutes would be ideal, one minute is better than zero minutes. When you're done, jot any comments in your journal.

Throughout your day and evening you can practice mindfulness. Pay attention as you pick up the remote. Focus on your breath for two minutes before eating breakfast (do you eat breakfast?). When you are grocery shopping, you can choose fruit or veggies mindfully. Yes, this takes more time than just grabbing and running on to the next task. During a meal, you might eat mindfully by paying attention to the food, paying attention as you chew, paying attention as you swallow. You might want to inform the people you are eating with before you engage in mindful eating! When you engage in house-cleaning tasks, you can do those tasks mindfully by paying attention as you do them. You can also be mindful as you walk, e.g., how various parts of your body move, how it feels when you transfer weight from one foot to the other. Notice if you are lost in thought, or if you are focusing on walking.

There are myriad ways to include mindfulness in your daily life. At first you'll probably have to remind yourself to be mindful. With practice, you may notice that you pay attention to the present moment more often. When you catch yourself worrying about something, or following inner dialog, you can gently bring your focus back to your breath in that moment. That can be an oasis, or a mini-vacation. You can write in your journal about mindfulness, including what it means to you and/or your experience of mindfulness.

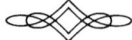

FIVE POSITIVE STATEMENTS

Far too many people could easily write five (or more) statements immediately about what's wrong with their body, their life, their job, their lack of a job, their home, etc. In this journal we're focusing on positive elements concerning you, your life, what you're thankful for. Remember that we're more likely to experience positive thoughts, gratitude, positive moods, and positive feelings when we focus on being positive. When we truly focus on something positive, there just isn't room to consider what's negative, even though there are negative features in everyone's life. So, the task is to write five statements about positive aspects of your body, yourself, your life, what you're thankful for, right in this present moment. You can write more than five statements, of course. If you find yourself writing the same five statements day after day, look for different positive aspects of yourself and your life, and what you're grateful for, to add to your list. Your positive statements could be "I have beautiful blue eyes" or "I enjoy petting my dog" or "I'm feeling calm and relaxed right now" or "I chuckle when I watch my grandson crawling across the carpet" or "I'm grateful for this beautiful sunny day."

How long did it take to come up with five original positive statements? How do you feel after writing those five positive statements? You can choose one statement to focus on during the day, or, if you're writing in your journal at night, you can focus on one positive statement as you get ready for bed. Focusing on one statement for awhile can set a tone for the upcoming day or sleep.

Another way to include positive statements in your journal is to write at the end of your day about positive things that occurred during that day, positive feelings or thoughts you experienced that day, things you're grateful for about that day. It's helpful to be thinking positive thoughts as you get ready for bed. Thinking positive thoughts at that time may help lead into peaceful sleep.

A few hints: Be sure to write about positive things in positive words. The statements "I have less pain today" or "I'm less depressed today" are NEGATIVE. They focus on pain and depression, respectively. This exercise is about positive statements. So, you might write about what you did today because you experienced less pain. For example, "I went to the movie this afternoon" can be either neutral or positive, while writing "I enjoyed going to the movie this afternoon" is positive. Going to the movie because you experienced less pain or less depression doesn't count. What counts is that you went out to the movie and you had a good time.

Focus on the present, today, right now. Your may write in your journal at night, reviewing the day. That's OK. Just be sure you are focusing on today. If something happened today that reminded you of something in the past, focus on today. If that thing in the past was positive, acknowledge it and bring that memory into your present awareness so you are happy now. For example, "Today's rain reminds me of dancing in the driveway in the pouring rain when I was five years old. I'm smiling as I remember that experience." That's positive!

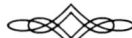

SELF RATING II
At the end of the day, or after writing your entries for that day in your journal, take a few seconds to note your current position on all four components of yourself: physiological, mental, emotional, spiritual. Use the same scale you used earlier. Rate quickly without thinking too much. Rate your immediate impression or awareness.

> *physiological:* your current level of physical comfort or relaxation
> *mental:* the quality of your current thoughts and mental preoccupation
> *emotional:* your feelings about your physical body, your thoughts, your life
> *spiritual:* your experience of connection with God/Goddess/Higher Self

The rating scale ranges from 1 to 7. Rate yourself on each of the four components.

1: totally uncomfortable; I experience no comfort or inner peace
2: a tiny amount of comfort or inner peace; I'm mostly aware of discomfort or disconnectedness
3: comfort or inner peace is somewhat overshadowed by discomfort or disconnectedness
4: my comfort or inner peace is balanced evenly with tension or disconnectedness
5: comfort or inner peace is slightly more noticeable than tension or disconnectedness
6: comfort or inner peace is predominant; I feel quite relaxed and peaceful
7: I'm totally relaxed and peaceful

After you've written in your journal for a couple of weeks, see if your second daily rating is different (hopefully, more positive) than your rating earlier in the day.

JOURNAL   **day # 1**

Circle today's day, then write the date and time:

SUNDAY   *MONDAY*   TUESDAY   WEDNESDAY   **THURSDAY**   FRIDAY   SATURDAY

DATE: TIME:

SELF RATING I (See page 5 for instructions and rating scale)

      physiological:

      mental:

      emotional:

      spiritual:

Notes:

Notes on the **BODY SCAN** exercise/meditation (See page 5 for instructions for the Body Scan)

Notes on **AWARENESS (INTERNAL/EXTERNAL)** (See page 8 for instructions on the Awareness exercise)

Notes on **EATING A RAISIN** (strawberry, walnut) (See page 10 for instructions on the Raisin (strawberry, walnut) Eating exercise)

Notes on **MINDFULNESS MEDITATION** (See page 10 for instructions on Mindfulness Meditation)

Notes on **FIVE POSITIVE STATEMENTS** (See page 11 for instructions on Five Positive Statements)

SELF RATING II (See page 12 for instructions and rating scale)

physiological:

mental:

emotional:

spiritual:

Notes:

JOURNAL   **day # 2**

Circle today's day, then write the date and time:

SUNDAY *MONDAY* TUESDAY WEDNESDAY **THURSDAY** FRIDAY SATURDAY

DATE: TIME:

SELF RATING I (See page 5 for instructions and rating scale)

physiological:

mental:

emotional:

spiritual:

Notes:

Notes on the **BODY SCAN** exercise/meditation (See page 5 for instructions for the Body Scan)

Notes on **AWARENESS (INTERNAL/EXTERNAL)** (See page 8 for instructions on the Awareness exercise)

Notes on **EATING A RAISIN** (strawberry, walnut) (See page 10 for instructions on the Raisin (strawberry, walnut) Eating exercise)

Notes on **MINDFULNESS MEDITATION** (See page 10 for instructions on Mindfulness Meditation)

Notes on **FIVE POSITIVE STATEMENTS** (See page 11 for instructions on Five Positive Statements)

SELF RATING II (See page 12 for instructions and rating scale)

    physiological:

    mental:

    emotional:

    spiritual:

Notes:

JOURNAL   **day # 3**

Circle today's day, then write the date and time:

SUNDAY *MONDAY* TUESDAY WEDNESDAY **THURSDAY** FRIDAY SATURDAY

DATE: TIME:

SELF RATING I (See page 5 for instructions and rating scale)

     physiological:

     mental:

     emotional:

     spiritual:

Notes:

Notes on the **BODY SCAN** exercise/meditation (See page 5 for instructions for the Body Scan)

Notes on **AWARENESS (INTERNAL/EXTERNAL)** (See page 8 for instructions on the Awareness exercise)

Notes on **EATING A RAISIN** (strawberry, walnut) (See page 10 for instructions on the Raisin (strawberry, walnut) Eating exercise)

Notes on **MINDFULNESS MEDITATION** (See page 10 for instructions on Mindfulness Meditation)

Notes on **FIVE POSITIVE STATEMENTS** (See page 11 for instructions on Five Positive Statements)

SELF RATING II (See page 12 for instructions and rating scale)

     physiological:

     mental:

     emotional:

     spiritual:

Notes:

JOURNAL   **day # 4**

Circle today's day, then write the date and time:

SUNDAY *MONDAY* TUESDAY WEDNESDAY **THURSDAY** FRIDAY SATURDAY

DATE: TIME:

SELF RATING I (See page 5 for instructions and rating scale)

    physiological:

    mental:

    emotional:

    spiritual:

Notes:

Notes on the **BODY SCAN** exercise/meditation (See page 5 for instructions for the Body Scan)

Notes on **AWARENESS (INTERNAL/EXTERNAL)** (See page 8 for instructions on the Awareness exercise)

Notes on **EATING A RAISIN** (strawberry, walnut) (See page 10 for instructions on the Raisin (strawberry, walnut) Eating exercise)

Notes on **MINDFULNESS MEDITATION** (See page 10 for instructions on Mindfulness Meditation)

Notes on **FIVE POSITIVE STATEMENTS** (See page 11 for instructions on Five Positive Statements)

SELF RATING II (See page 12 for instructions and rating scale)

    physiological:

    mental:

    emotional:

    spiritual:

Notes:

JOURNAL   **day # 5**

Circle today's day, then write the date and time:

SUNDAY *MONDAY* TUESDAY WEDNESDAY **THURSDAY** FRIDAY SATURDAY

DATE: TIME:

SELF RATING I (See page 5 for instructions and rating scale)

      physiological:

      mental:

      emotional:

      spiritual:

Notes:

Notes on the **BODY SCAN** exercise/meditation (See page 5 for instructions for the Body Scan)

Notes on **AWARENESS (INTERNAL/EXTERNAL)** (See page 8 for instructions on the Awareness exercise)

Notes on **EATING A RAISIN** (strawberry, walnut) (See page 10 for instructions on the Raisin (strawberry, walnut) Eating exercise)

Notes on **MINDFULNESS MEDITATION** (See page 10 for instructions on Mindfulness Meditation)

Notes on **FIVE POSITIVE STATEMENTS** (See page 11 for instructions on Five Positive Statements)

SELF RATING II (See page 12 for instructions and rating scale)

    physiological:

    mental:

    emotional:

    spiritual:

Notes:

JOURNAL   **day # 6**

Circle today's day, then write the date and time:

SUNDAY *MONDAY* TUESDAY WEDNESDAY **THURSDAY** FRIDAY SATURDAY

DATE: TIME:

SELF RATING I (See page 5 for instructions and rating scale)

     physiological:

     mental:

     emotional:

     spiritual:

Notes:

Notes on the **BODY SCAN** exercise/meditation (See page 5 for instructions for the Body Scan)

Notes on **AWARENESS (INTERNAL/EXTERNAL)** (See page 8 for instructions on the Awareness exercise)

Notes on **EATING A RAISIN** (strawberry, walnut) (See page 10 for instructions on the Raisin (strawberry, walnut) Eating exercise)

Notes on **MINDFULNESS MEDITATION** (See page 10 for instructions on Mindfulness Meditation)

Notes on **FIVE POSITIVE STATEMENTS** (See page 11 for instructions on Five Positive Statements)

SELF RATING II (See page 12 for instructions and rating scale)

      physiological:

      mental:

      emotional:

      spiritual:

Notes:

JOURNAL   **day # 7**

Circle today's day, then write the date and time:

SUNDAY *MONDAY* TUESDAY   WEDNESDAY **THURSDAY**   FRIDAY   SATURDAY

DATE: TIME:

SELF RATING I (See page 5 for instructions and rating scale)

  physiological:

  mental:

  emotional:

  spiritual:

Notes:

Notes on the **BODY SCAN** exercise/meditation (See page 5 for instructions for the Body Scan)

Notes on **AWARENESS (INTERNAL/EXTERNAL)** (See page 8 for instructions on the Awareness exercise)

Notes on **EATING A RAISIN** (strawberry, walnut) (See page 10 for instructions on the Raisin (strawberry, walnut) Eating exercise)

Notes on **MINDFULNESS MEDITATION** (See page 10 for instructions on Mindfulness Meditation)

Notes on **FIVE POSITIVE STATEMENTS** (See page 11 for instructions on Five Positive Statements)

SELF RATING II (See page 12 for instructions and rating scale)

     physiological:

     mental:

     emotional:

     spiritual:

Notes:

JOURNAL   **day # 8**

Circle today's day, then write the date and time:

SUNDAY   *MONDAY*   TUESDAY   WEDNESDAY   **THURSDAY**   FRIDAY   SATURDAY

DATE: TIME:

SELF RATING I (See page 5 for instructions and rating scale)

     physiological:

     mental:

     emotional:

     spiritual:

Notes:

Notes on the **BODY SCAN** exercise/meditation (See page 5 for instructions for the Body Scan)

Notes on **AWARENESS (INTERNAL/EXTERNAL)** (See page 8 for instructions on the Awareness exercise)

Notes on **EATING A RAISIN** (strawberry, walnut) (See page 10 for instructions on the Raisin (strawberry, walnut) Eating exercise)

Notes on **MINDFULNESS MEDITATION** (See page 10 for instructions on Mindfulness Meditation)

Notes on **FIVE POSITIVE STATEMENTS** (See page 11 for instructions on Five Positive Statements)

SELF RATING II (See page 12 for instructions and rating scale)

      physiological:

      mental:

      emotional:

      spiritual:

Notes:

JOURNAL   **day # 9**

Circle today's day, then write the date and time:

SUNDAY *MONDAY* TUESDAY WEDNESDAY **THURSDAY** FRIDAY SATURDAY

DATE: TIME:

SELF RATING I (See page 5 for instructions and rating scale)

> physiological:
>
> mental:
>
> emotional:
>
> spiritual:

Notes:

Notes on the **BODY SCAN** exercise/meditation (See page 5 for instructions for the Body Scan)

Notes on **AWARENESS (INTERNAL/EXTERNAL)** (See page 8 for instructions on the Awareness exercise)

Notes on **EATING A RAISIN** (strawberry, walnut) (See page 10 for instructions on the Raisin (strawberry, walnut) Eating exercise)

Notes on **MINDFULNESS MEDITATION** (See page 10 for instructions on Mindfulness Meditation)

Notes on **FIVE POSITIVE STATEMENTS** (See page 11 for instructions on Five Positive Statements)

SELF RATING II (See page 12 for instructions and rating scale)

    physiological:

    mental:

    emotional:

    spiritual:

Notes:

JOURNAL   **day # 10**

Circle today's day, then write the date and time:

SUNDAY *MONDAY* TUESDAY WEDNESDAY **THURSDAY** FRIDAY SATURDAY

DATE: TIME:

SELF RATING I (See page 5 for instructions and rating scale)

    physiological:

    mental:

    emotional:

    spiritual:

Notes:

Notes on the **BODY SCAN** exercise/meditation (See page 5 for instructions for the Body Scan)

Notes on **AWARENESS (INTERNAL/EXTERNAL)** (See page 8 for instructions on the Awareness exercise)

Notes on **EATING A RAISIN** (strawberry, walnut) (See page 10 for instructions on the Raisin (strawberry, walnut) Eating exercise)

Notes on **MINDFULNESS MEDITATION** (See page 10 for instructions on Mindfulness Meditation)

Notes on **FIVE POSITIVE STATEMENTS** (See page 11 for instructions on Five Positive Statements)

SELF RATING II (See page 12 for instructions and rating scale)

      physiological:

      mental:

      emotional:

      spiritual:

Notes:

JOURNAL **day # 11**

Circle today's day, then write the date and time:

SUNDAY *MONDAY* TUESDAY WEDNESDAY **THURSDAY** FRIDAY SATURDAY

DATE: TIME:

SELF RATING I (See page 5 for instructions and rating scale)

physiological:

mental:

emotional:

spiritual:

Notes:

Notes on the **BODY SCAN** exercise/meditation (See page 5 for instructions for the Body Scan)

Notes on **AWARENESS (INTERNAL/EXTERNAL)** (See page 8 for instructions on the Awareness exercise)

Notes on **EATING A RAISIN** (strawberry, walnut) (See page 10 for instructions on the Raisin (strawberry, walnut) Eating exercise)

Notes on **MINDFULNESS MEDITATION** (See page 10 for instructions on Mindfulness Meditation)

Notes on **FIVE POSITIVE STATEMENTS** (See page 11 for instructions on Five Positive Statements)

SELF RATING II (See page 12 for instructions and rating scale)

      physiological:

      mental:

      emotional:

      spiritual:

Notes:

JOURNAL day # 12

Circle today's day, then write the date and time:

SUNDAY *monday* TUESDAY WEDNESDAY **THURSDAY** FRIDAY SATURDAY

DATE: TIME:

SELF RATING I (See page 5 for instructions and rating scale)

physiological:

mental:

emotional:

spiritual:

Notes:

Notes on the **BODY SCAN** exercise/meditation (See page 5 for instructions for the Body Scan)

Notes on **AWARENESS (INTERNAL/EXTERNAL)** (See page 8 for instructions on the Awareness exercise)

Notes on **EATING A RAISIN** (strawberry, walnut) (See page 10 for instructions on the Raisin (strawberry, walnut) Eating exercise)

Notes on **MINDFULNESS MEDITATION** (See page 10 for instructions on Mindfulness Meditation)

Notes on **FIVE POSITIVE STATEMENTS** (See page 11 for instructions on Five Positive Statements)

SELF RATING II (See page 12 for instructions and rating scale)

     physiological:

     mental:

     emotional:

     spiritual:

Notes:

JOURNAL   **day # 13**

Circle today's day, then write the date and time:

SUNDAY *MONDAY* TUESDAY WEDNESDAY THURSDAY FRIDAY SATURDAY

DATE: TIME:

SELF RATING I (See page 5 for instructions and rating scale)

      physiological:

      mental:

      emotional:

      spiritual:

Notes:

Notes on the **BODY SCAN** exercise/meditation (See page 5 for instructions for the Body Scan)

Notes on **AWARENESS (INTERNAL/EXTERNAL)** (See page 8 for instructions on the Awareness exercise)

Notes on **EATING A RAISIN** (strawberry, walnut) (See page 10 for instructions on the Raisin (strawberry, walnut) Eating exercise)

Notes on **MINDFULNESS MEDITATION** (See page 10 for instructions on Mindfulness Meditation)

Notes on **FIVE POSITIVE STATEMENTS** (See page 11 for instructions on Five Positive Statements)

SELF RATING II (See page 12 for instructions and rating scale)

     physiological:

     mental:

     emotional:

     spiritual:

Notes:

JOURNAL   **day # 14**

Circle today's day, then write the date and time:

SUNDAY   *MONDAY*   TUESDAY   WEDNESDAY   **THURSDAY**   FRIDAY   SATURDAY

DATE: TIME:

SELF RATING I (See page 5 for instructions and rating scale)

      physiological:

      mental:

      emotional:

      spiritual:

Notes:

Notes on the **BODY SCAN** exercise/meditation (See page 5 for instructions for the Body Scan)

Notes on **AWARENESS (INTERNAL/EXTERNAL)** (See page 8 for instructions on the Awareness exercise)

Notes on **EATING A RAISIN** (strawberry, walnut) (See page 10 for instructions on the Raisin (strawberry, walnut) Eating exercise)

Notes on **MINDFULNESS MEDITATION** (See page 10 for instructions on Mindfulness Meditation)

Notes on **FIVE POSITIVE STATEMENTS** (See page 11 for instructions on Five Positive Statements)

SELF RATING II (See page 12 for instructions and rating scale)

      physiological:

      mental:

      emotional:

      spiritual:

Notes:

JOURNAL   **day # 15**

Circle today's day, then write the date and time:

SUNDAY *MONDAY* TUESDAY WEDNESDAY THURSDAY FRIDAY SATURDAY

DATE: TIME:

SELF RATING I (See page 5 for instructions and rating scale)

     physiological:

     mental:

     emotional:

     spiritual:

Notes:

Notes on the **BODY SCAN** exercise/meditation (See page 5 for instructions for the Body Scan)

Notes on **AWARENESS (INTERNAL/EXTERNAL)** (See page 8 for instructions on the Awareness exercise)

Notes on **EATING A RAISIN** (strawberry, walnut) (See page 10 for instructions on the Raisin (strawberry, walnut) Eating exercise)

Notes on **MINDFULNESS MEDITATION** (See page 10 for instructions on Mindfulness Meditation)

Notes on **FIVE POSITIVE STATEMENTS** (See page 11 for instructions on Five Positive Statements)

SELF RATING II (See page 12 for instructions and rating scale)

    physiological:

    mental:

    emotional:

    spiritual:

Notes::

JOURNAL   **day # 16**

Circle today's day, then write the date and time:

SUNDAY *MONDAY* TUESDAY WEDNESDAY **THURSDAY** FRIDAY SATURDAY

DATE: TIME:

SELF RATING I (See page 5 for instructions and rating scale)

    physiological:

    mental:

    emotional:

    spiritual:

Notes:

Notes on the **BODY SCAN** exercise/meditation (See page 5 for instructions for the Body Scan)

Notes on **AWARENESS (INTERNAL/EXTERNAL)** (See page 8 for instructions on the Awareness exercise)

Notes on **EATING A RAISIN** (strawberry, walnut) (See page 10 for instructions on the Raisin (strawberry, walnut) Eating exercise)

Notes on **MINDFULNESS MEDITATION** (See page 10 for instructions on Mindfulness Meditation)

Notes on **FIVE POSITIVE STATEMENTS** (See page 11 for instructions on Five Positive Statements)

SELF RATING II (See page 12 for instructions and rating scale)

      physiological:

      mental:

      emotional:

      spiritual:

Notes:

JOURNAL   **day # 17**

Circle today's day, then write the date and time:

SUNDAY *MONDAY* TUESDAY WEDNESDAY **THURSDAY** FRIDAY SATURDAY

DATE: TIME:

SELF RATING I (See page 5 for instructions and rating scale)

     physiological:

     mental:

     emotional:

     spiritual:

Notes:

Notes on the **BODY SCAN** exercise/meditation (See page 5 for instructions for the Body Scan)

Notes on **AWARENESS (INTERNAL/EXTERNAL)** (See page 8 for instructions on the Awareness exercise)

Notes on **EATING A RAISIN** (strawberry, walnut) (See page 10 for instructions on the Raisin (strawberry, walnut) Eating exercise)

Notes on **MINDFULNESS MEDITATION** (See page 10 for instructions on Mindfulness Meditation)

Notes on **FIVE POSITIVE STATEMENTS** (See page 11 for instructions on Five Positive Statements)

SELF RATING II (See page 12 for instructions and rating scale)

      physiological:

      mental:

      emotional:

      spiritual:

Notes:

JOURNAL   **day # 18**

Circle today's day, then write the date and time:

SUNDAY *MONDAY* TUESDAY WEDNESDAY THURSDAY FRIDAY SATURDAY

DATE: TIME:

SELF RATING I (See page 5 for instructions and rating scale)

     physiological:

     mental:

     emotional:

     spiritual:

Notes:

Notes on the **BODY SCAN** exercise/meditation (See page 5 for instructions for the Body Scan)

Notes on **AWARENESS (INTERNAL/EXTERNAL)** (See page 8 for instructions on the Awareness exercise)

Notes on **EATING A RAISIN** (strawberry, walnut) (See page 10 for instructions on the Raisin (strawberry, walnut) Eating exercise)

Notes on **MINDFULNESS MEDITATION** (See page 10 for instructions on Mindfulness Meditation)

Notes on **FIVE POSITIVE STATEMENTS** (See page 11 for instructions on Five Positive Statements)

SELF RATING II (See page 12 for instructions and rating scale)

    physiological:

    mental:

    emotional:

    spiritual:

Notes:

JOURNAL   **day # 19**

Circle today's day, then write the date and time:

SUNDAY   *MONDAY*   TUESDAY   WEDNESDAY   THURSDAY   FRIDAY   SATURDAY

DATE: TIME:

SELF RATING I (See page 5 for instructions and rating scale)

      physiological:

      mental:

      emotional:

      spiritual:

Notes:

Notes on the **BODY SCAN** exercise/meditation (See page 5 for instructions for the Body Scan)

Notes on **AWARENESS (INTERNAL/EXTERNAL)** (See page 8 for instructions on the Awareness exercise)

Notes on **EATING A RAISIN** (strawberry, walnut) (See page 10 for instructions on the Raisin (strawberry, walnut) Eating exercise)

Notes on **MINDFULNESS MEDITATION** (See page 10 for instructions on Mindfulness Meditation)

Notes on **FIVE POSITIVE STATEMENTS** (See page 11 for instructions on Five Positive Statements)

SELF RATING II (See page 12 for instructions and rating scale)

     physiological:

     mental:

     emotional:

     spiritual:

Notes:

JOURNAL   **day # 20**

Circle today's day, then write the date and time:

SUNDAY   *MONDAY*   TUESDAY   WEDNESDAY   THURSDAY   FRIDAY   SATURDAY

DATE: TIME:

SELF RATING I (See page 5 for instructions and rating scale)

      physiological:

      mental:

      emotional:

      spiritual:

Notes:

Notes on the **BODY SCAN** exercise/meditation (See page 5 for instructions for the Body Scan)

Notes on **AWARENESS (INTERNAL/EXTERNAL)** (See page 8 for instructions on the Awareness exercise)

Notes on **EATING A RAISIN** (strawberry, walnut) (See page 10 for instructions on the Raisin (strawberry, walnut) Eating exercise)

Notes on **MINDFULNESS MEDITATION** (See page 10 for instructions on Mindfulness Meditation)

Notes on **FIVE POSITIVE STATEMENTS** (See page 11 for instructions on Five Positive Statements)

SELF RATING II (See page 12 for instructions and rating scale)

     physiological:

     mental:

     emotional:

     spiritual:

Notes:

JOURNAL   **day # 21**

Circle today's day, then write the date and time:

SUNDAY *MONDAY* TUESDAY   WEDNESDAY THURSDAY   FRIDAY   SATURDAY

DATE: TIME:

SELF RATING I (See page 5 for instructions and rating scale)

     physiological:

     mental:

     emotional:

     spiritual:

Notes:

Notes on the **BODY SCAN** exercise/meditation (See page 5 for instructions for the Body Scan)

Notes on **AWARENESS (INTERNAL/EXTERNAL)** (See page 8 for instructions on the Awareness exercise)

Notes on **EATING A RAISIN** (strawberry, walnut) (See page 10 for instructions on the Raisin (strawberry, walnut) Eating exercise)

Notes on **MINDFULNESS MEDITATION** (See page 10 for instructions on Mindfulness Meditation)

Notes on **FIVE POSITIVE STATEMENTS** (See page 11 for instructions on Five Positive Statements)

SELF RATING II (See page 12 for instructions and rating scale)

      physiological:

      mental:

      emotional:

      spiritual:

Notes:

JOURNAL   **day # 22**

Circle today's day, then write the date and time:

SUNDAY *MONDAY* TUESDAY WEDNESDAY **THURSDAY** FRIDAY SATURDAY

DATE: TIME:

SELF RATING I (See page 5 for instructions and rating scale)

     physiological:

     mental:

     emotional:

     spiritual:

Notes:

Notes on the **BODY SCAN** exercise/meditation (See page 5 for instructions for the Body Scan)

Notes on **AWARENESS (INTERNAL/EXTERNAL)** (See page 8 for instructions on the Awareness exercise)

Notes on **EATING A RAISIN** (strawberry, walnut) (See page 10 for instructions on the Raisin (strawberry, walnut) Eating exercise)

Notes on **MINDFULNESS MEDITATION** (See page 10 for instructions on Mindfulness Meditation)

Notes on **FIVE POSITIVE STATEMENTS** (See page 11 for instructions on Five Positive Statements)

SELF RATING II (See page 12 for instructions and rating scale)

    physiological:

    mental:

    emotional:

    spiritual:

Notes:

JOURNAL   **day # 23**

Circle today's day, then write the date and time:

SUNDAY *MONDAY* TUESDAY WEDNESDAY **THURSDAY** FRIDAY SATURDAY

DATE: TIME:

SELF RATING I (See page 5 for instructions and rating scale)

> physiological:
>
> mental:
>
> emotional:
>
> spiritual:

Notes:

Notes on the **BODY SCAN** exercise/meditation (See page 5 for instructions for the Body Scan)

Notes on **AWARENESS (INTERNAL/EXTERNAL)** (See page 8 for instructions on the Awareness exercise)

Notes on **EATING A RAISIN** (strawberry, walnut) (See page 10 for instructions on the Raisin (strawberry, walnut) Eating exercise)

Notes on **MINDFULNESS MEDITATION** (See page 10 for instructions on Mindfulness Meditation)

Notes on **FIVE POSITIVE STATEMENTS** (See page 11 for instructions on Five Positive Statements)

SELF RATING II (See page 12 for instructions and rating scale)

     physiological:

     mental:

     emotional:

     spiritual:

Notes:

JOURNAL   **day # 24**

Circle today's day, then write the date and time:

SUNDAY *MONDAY* TUESDAY WEDNESDAY **THURSDAY** FRIDAY SATURDAY

DATE: TIME:

SELF RATING I (See page 5 for instructions and rating scale)

    physiological:

    mental:

    emotional:

    spiritual:

Notes:

Notes on the **BODY SCAN** exercise/meditation (See page 5 for instructions for the Body Scan)

Notes on **AWARENESS (INTERNAL/EXTERNAL)** (See page 8 for instructions on the Awareness exercise)

Notes on **EATING A RAISIN** (strawberry, walnut) (See page 10 for instructions on the Raisin (strawberry, walnut) Eating exercise)

Notes on **MINDFULNESS MEDITATION** (See page 10 for instructions on Mindfulness Meditation)

Notes on **FIVE POSITIVE STATEMENTS** (See page 11 for instructions on Five Positive Statements)

SELF RATING II (See page 12 for instructions and rating scale)

       physiological:

       mental:

       emotional:

       spiritual:

Notes:

JOURNAL   **day # 25**

Circle today's day, then write the date and time:

SUNDAY *MONDAY* TUESDAY WEDNESDAY THURSDAY FRIDAY SATURDAY

DATE: TIME:

SELF RATING I (See page 5 for instructions and rating scale)

     physiological:

     mental:

     emotional:

     spiritual:

Notes:

Notes on the **BODY SCAN** exercise/meditation (See page 5 for instructions for the Body Scan)

Notes on **AWARENESS (INTERNAL/EXTERNAL)** (See page 8 for instructions on the Awareness exercise)

Notes on **EATING A RAISIN** (strawberry, walnut) (See page 10 for instructions on the Raisin (strawberry, walnut) Eating exercise)

Notes on **MINDFULNESS MEDITATION** (See page 10 for instructions on Mindfulness Meditation)

Notes on **FIVE POSITIVE STATEMENTS** (See page 11 for instructions on Five Positive Statements)

SELF RATING II (See page 12 for instructions and rating scale)

 physiological:

 mental:

 emotional:

 spiritual:

Notes:

JOURNAL   **day # 26**

Circle today's day, then write the date and time:

SUNDAY *MONDAY* TUESDAY WEDNESDAY **THURSDAY** FRIDAY SATURDAY

DATE: TIME:

SELF RATING I (See page 5 for instructions and rating scale)

    physiological:

    mental:

    emotional:

    spiritual:

Notes:

Notes on the **BODY SCAN** exercise/meditation (See page 5 for instructions for the Body Scan)

Notes on **AWARENESS (INTERNAL/EXTERNAL)** (See page 8 for instructions on the Awareness exercise)

Notes on **EATING A RAISIN** (strawberry, walnut) (See page 10 for instructions on the Raisin (strawberry, walnut) Eating exercise)

Notes on **MINDFULNESS MEDITATION** (See page 10 for instructions on Mindfulness Meditation)

Notes on **FIVE POSITIVE STATEMENTS** (See page 11 for instructions on Five Positive Statements)

SELF RATING II (See page 12 for instructions and rating scale)

    physiological:

    mental:

    emotional:

    spiritual:

Notes:

JOURNAL   **day # 27**

Circle today's day, then write the date and time:

SUNDAY *MONDAY* TUESDAY WEDNESDAY **THURSDAY** FRIDAY SATURDAY

DATE: TIME:

SELF RATING I (See page 5 for instructions and rating scale)

       physiological:

       mental:

       emotional:

       spiritual:

Notes:

Notes on the **BODY SCAN** exercise/meditation (See page 5 for instructions for the Body Scan)

Notes on **AWARENESS (INTERNAL/EXTERNAL)** (See page 8 for instructions on the Awareness exercise)

Notes on **EATING A RAISIN** (strawberry, walnut) (See page 10 for instructions on the Raisin (strawberry, walnut) Eating exercise)

Notes on **MINDFULNESS MEDITATION** (See page 10 for instructions on Mindfulness Meditation)

Notes on **FIVE POSITIVE STATEMENTS** (See page 11 for instructions on Five Positive Statements)

SELF RATING II (See page 12 for instructions and rating scale)

      physiological:

      mental:

      emotional:

      spiritual:

Notes:

JOURNAL   **day # 28**

Circle today's day, then write the date and time:

SUNDAY *MONDAY* TUESDAY WEDNESDAY **THURSDAY** FRIDAY SATURDAY

DATE: TIME:

SELF RATING I (See page 5 for instructions and rating scale)

     physiological:

     mental:

     emotional:

     spiritual:

Notes:

Notes on the **BODY SCAN** exercise/meditation (See page 5 for instructions for the Body Scan)

Notes on **AWARENESS (INTERNAL/EXTERNAL)** (See page 8 for instructions on the Awareness exercise)

Notes on **EATING A RAISIN** (strawberry, walnut) (See page 10 for instructions on the Raisin (strawberry, walnut) Eating exercise)

Notes on **MINDFULNESS MEDITATION** (See page 10 for instructions on Mindfulness Meditation)

Notes on **FIVE POSITIVE STATEMENTS** (See page 11 for instructions on Five Positive Statements)

SELF RATING II (See page 12 for instructions and rating scale)

    physiological:

    mental:

    emotional:

    spiritual:

Notes:

JOURNAL   **day # 29**

Circle today's day, then write the date and time:

SUNDAY *MONDAY* TUESDAY WEDNESDAY THURSDAY FRIDAY SATURDAY

DATE: TIME:

SELF RATING I (See page 5 for instructions and rating scale)

     physiological:

     mental:

     emotional:

     spiritual:

Notes:

Notes on the **BODY SCAN** exercise/meditation (See page 5 for instructions for the Body Scan)

Notes on **AWARENESS (INTERNAL/EXTERNAL)** (See page 8 for instructions on the Awareness exercise)

Notes on **EATING A RAISIN** (strawberry, walnut) (See page 10 for instructions on the Raisin (strawberry, walnut) Eating exercise)

Notes on **MINDFULNESS MEDITATION** (See page 10 for instructions on Mindfulness Meditation)

Notes on **FIVE POSITIVE STATEMENTS** (See page 11 for instructions on Five Positive Statements)

SELF RATING II (See page 12 for instructions and rating scale)

     physiological:

     mental:

     emotional:

     spiritual:

Notes:

JOURNAL **day # 30**

Circle today's day, then write the date and time:

SUNDAY *MONDAY* TUESDAY WEDNESDAY **THURSDAY** FRIDAY SATURDAY

DATE: TIME:

SELF RATING I (See page 5 for instructions and rating scale)

    physiological:

    mental:

    emotional:

    spiritual:

Notes:

Notes on the **BODY SCAN** exercise/meditation (See page 5 for instructions for the Body Scan)

Notes on **AWARENESS (INTERNAL/EXTERNAL)** (See page 8 for instructions on the Awareness exercise)

Notes on **EATING A RAISIN** (strawberry, walnut) (See page 10 for instructions on the Raisin (strawberry, walnut) Eating exercise)

Notes on **MINDFULNESS MEDITATION** (See page 10 for instructions on Mindfulness Meditation)

Notes on **FIVE POSITIVE STATEMENTS** (See page 11 for instructions on Five Positive Statements)

SELF RATING II (See page 12 for instructions and rating scale)

    physiological:

    mental:

    emotional:

    spiritual:

Notes:

FINAL THOUGHTS AND ENCOURAGEMENT

Creating meaningful change usually takes courage, time, and persistent effort. Time alone isn't sufficient; it's time filled with practice that counts most. Even if you have courage, persistent practice, and lots of positive reinforcement from loved ones and your health care providers, it's possible to feel that you aren't making progress fast enough, or to fall into a "slump." The best athletes can fall into a slump, yet they work their way out of them step by step (without resorting to using performance enhancing drugs). I encourage you to do the same.

A period of negativity or a slump may be punctuated by questions and statements such as "why am I bothering to do these exercises?" or "I'd rather do XYZ than these exercises" or "I don't have time; I'll do the exercises tomorrow." If any of these statements sounds like you, you might review your goals to see if they are still important to you. If the goals aren't important any more, you can write new goals, or stop pursuing these exercises until you become motivated enough to re-start the exercises.

You might be affected by "approach/avoidance." You may have been drawn initially towards your goal by motivation, desire to feel better, following your practitioner's suggestions, etc. That is the "approach." "Avoidance" often appears when we discover how much work it takes to reach the goal, or we perceive a negative aspect to our goal that detracts from our initial drive to move forward toward it. It can help to focus on positive qualities of your goal, re-affirming your commitment to reaching your goal, talking positively to yourself about the value of "baby steps" toward your goal.

Responsibility is a key issue. Own your decisions, whether that decision is to continue working toward your goal, or whether that decision is to change your goal, to take a respite or to quit altogether. Our power usually lies in the choices we make.

See if there is a pattern in your current behavior or thoughts. Are you re-playing an old theme? It could be a theme like "it's too hard" or "I'm not good enough" or "I'm scared that XXX will happen if I succeed." Do you expect too much of yourself too fast, and then berate yourself for being normal? You can explore your theme on your own, or discuss your pattern with a qualified professional.

Lasting change takes repeated effort, time, patience, and a sense of self worth. I encourage you to stay on your positive path. It's worth it, and you are, too.

REFERENCES

Childre, D. & Rozman, D. (2003). *Transforming Anger.* Oakland, CA: New Harbinger.

Childre, D. & Rozman, D. (2005). *Transforming Stress.* Oakland, CA: New Harbinger.

Davis, M., Eshelman, E. R., & McKay, M. (1995). *The Relaxation & Stress Reduction Workbook, Fourth Edition.* Oakland, CA: New Harbinger.

Hendricks, G. (1995). *Conscious Breathing.* New York: Bantam Books.

Munoz, R. F., Beardslee, W. R., & Leykin, Y. (2012). Major Depression Can Be Prevented. *American Psychologist, 67(4),* 285-295.

Kabat-Zinn, J. (1990). *Full Catastrophe Living: Using the Wisdom of Your Body and Mind to Face Stress, Pain, and Illness.* New York: Delta.

Kabat-Zinn, J. (1994). *Wherever You Go There You Are: Mindfulness meditation in everyday life.* New York: Hyperion.

Lipton, B. (2005). *The Biology of Belief.* Santa Rosa, CA: Mountain of Love/Elite Books.

National Research Council & Institute of Medicine (2009). *Preventing mental, emotional, and behavioral disorders among young people: Progress and possibilities* (M. E. O'Connell, T. Boat, & K. E. Warner, Eds.). Washington, D.C.: National Academies Press.

Preston, J. (1989). *You Can Beat Depression.* San Luis Obispo, CA: Impact Publishers.

Seligman, M. E. P. (2002). *Authentic Happiness.* New York: Free Press.

Yapko, M. (2011). *Mindfulness and Hypnosis: the power of suggestion to transform experience.* New York: W. W. Norton.

CPSIA information can be obtained at www.ICGtesting.com
Printed in the USA
LVOW09s1144310813

350424LV00008B/291/P